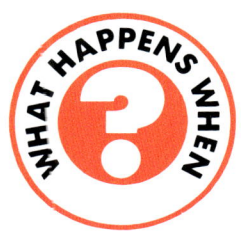

WHAT HAPPENS WHEN **?**

What happens when
People
Talk?

Daphne Butler

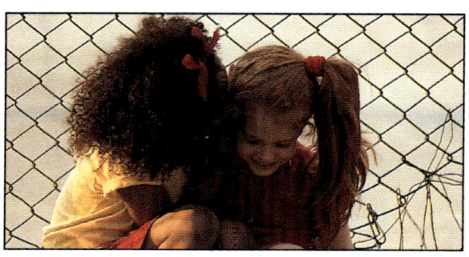

SIMON & SCHUSTER
YOUNG BOOKS

This book was conceived for
Simon & Schuster Young Books by
Globe Enterprises of Nantwich, Cheshire

Design: SPL Design
Photographs: Zefa

First published in Great Britain in 1993
by Simon & Schuster Young Books
Campus 400, Maylands Avenue
Hemel Hempstead, Herts HP2 7EZ

© 1993 Globe Enterprises

Printed and bound in Singapore
by Kim Hup Lee Printing Co Pte Ltd

A catalogue record for this book is available
from the British Library
ISBN 0 7500 1288 9

Contents

Making a noise

When you were born one of the first things you did was to fill your lungs with air and to cry.

You had learnt your first lesson— how to communicate by making a noise.

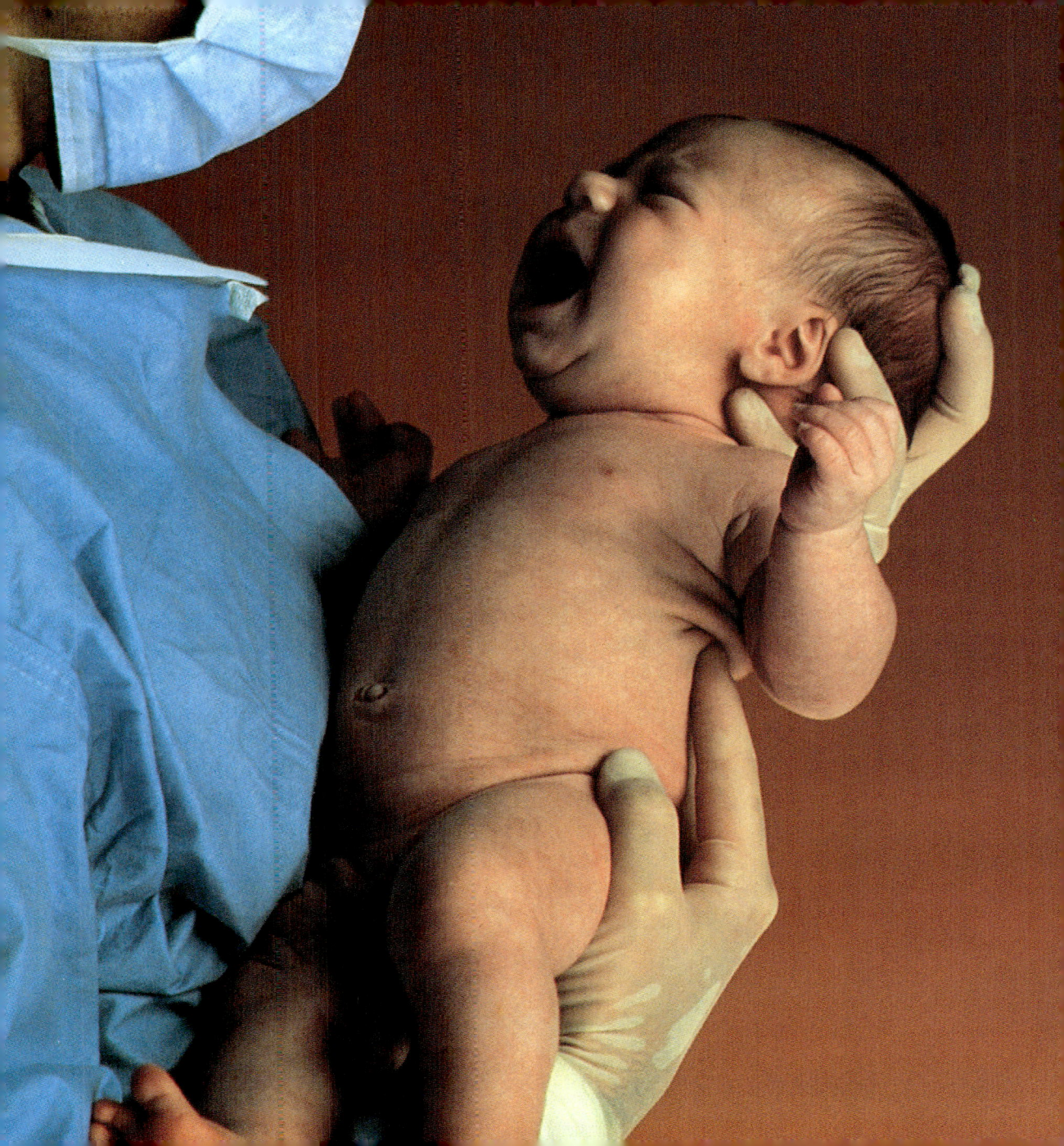

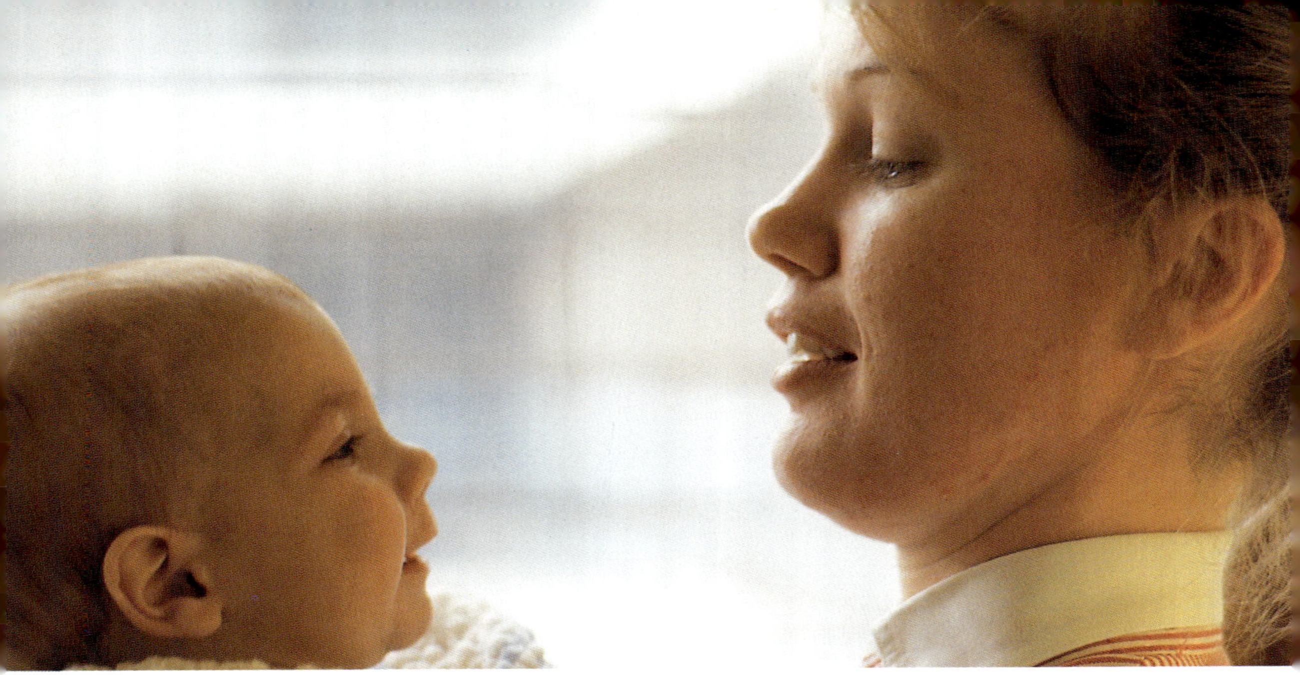

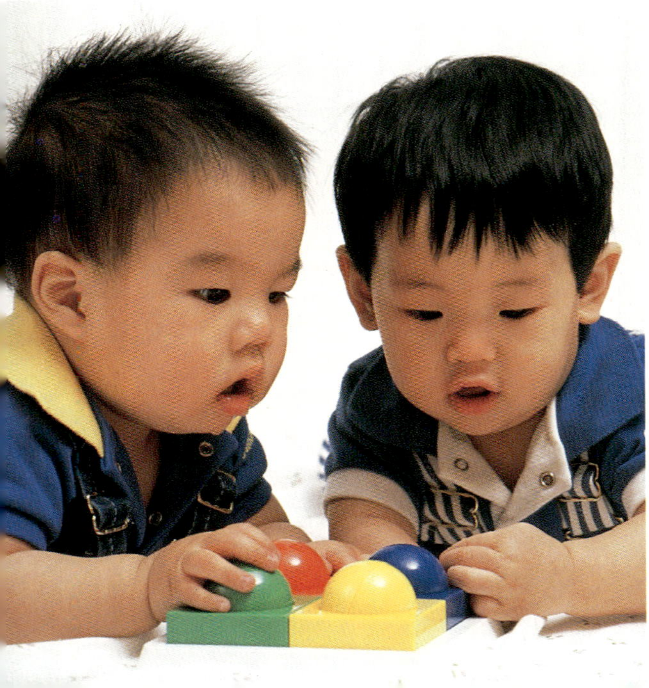

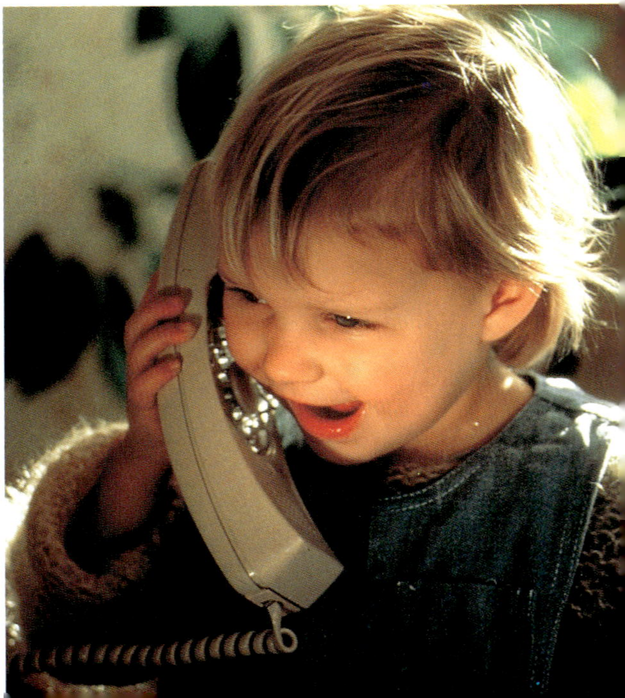

Listening and copying

As you grew, you listened to the people around you. At first, the sounds meant nothing to you.

Then, slowly you began to understand simple words like 'bath' and 'dinner' and 'bedtime'.

By listening and copying, you learnt to make the sounds yourself. By the time you were two years old, you had probably started to talk.

9

What makes sound?

If you put your hand on your throat while you are talking, you will feel your throat vibrating.

Inside there is a voice box.
It vibrates when air passes through and the vibrations make sound.

You can talk because muscles change the shape of your voice box to make different sounds.

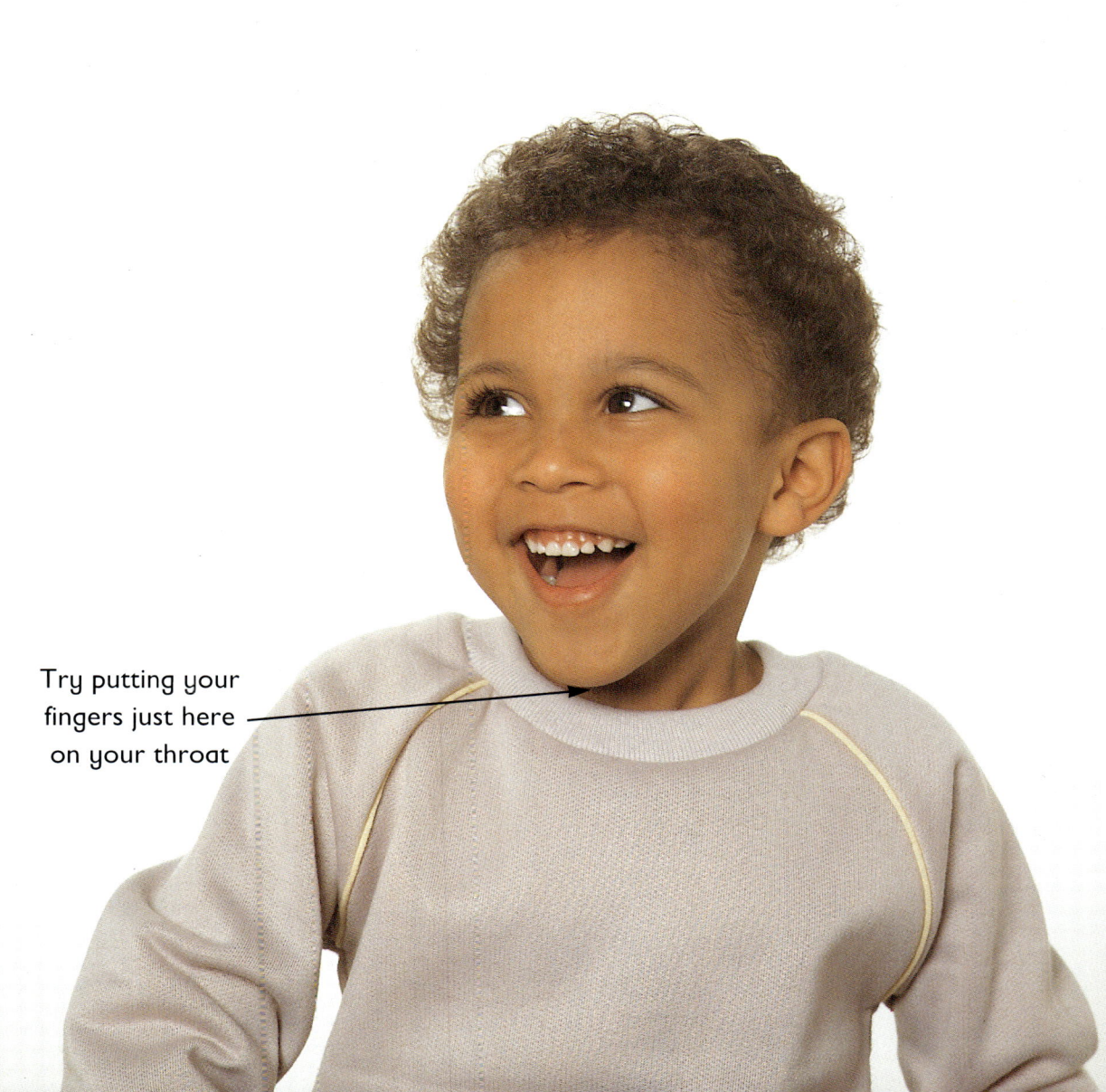

Try putting your
fingers just here
on your throat

Questions and answers

Once you can talk you can both ask, and answer, questions.

Through talking, you learn more and more about the world around you day by day.

12

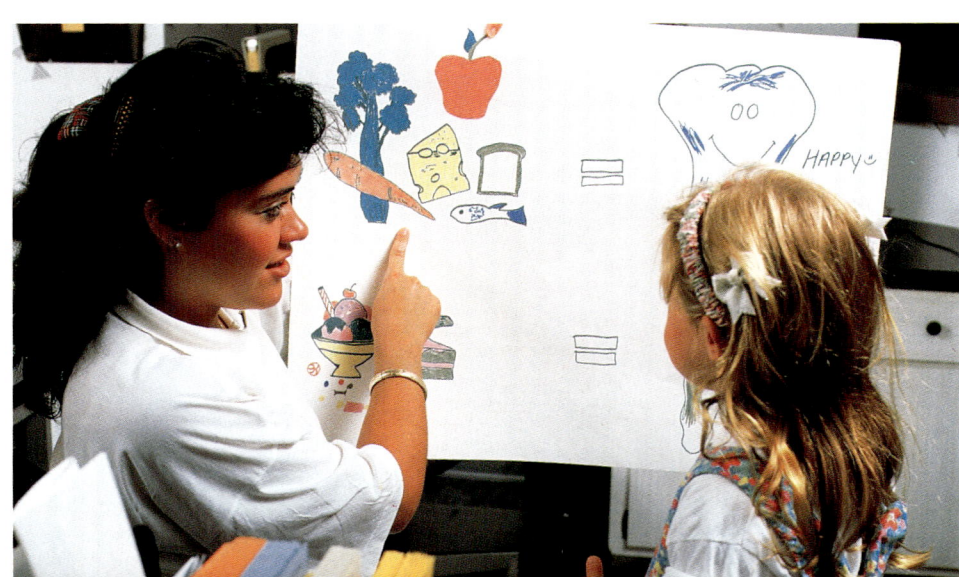

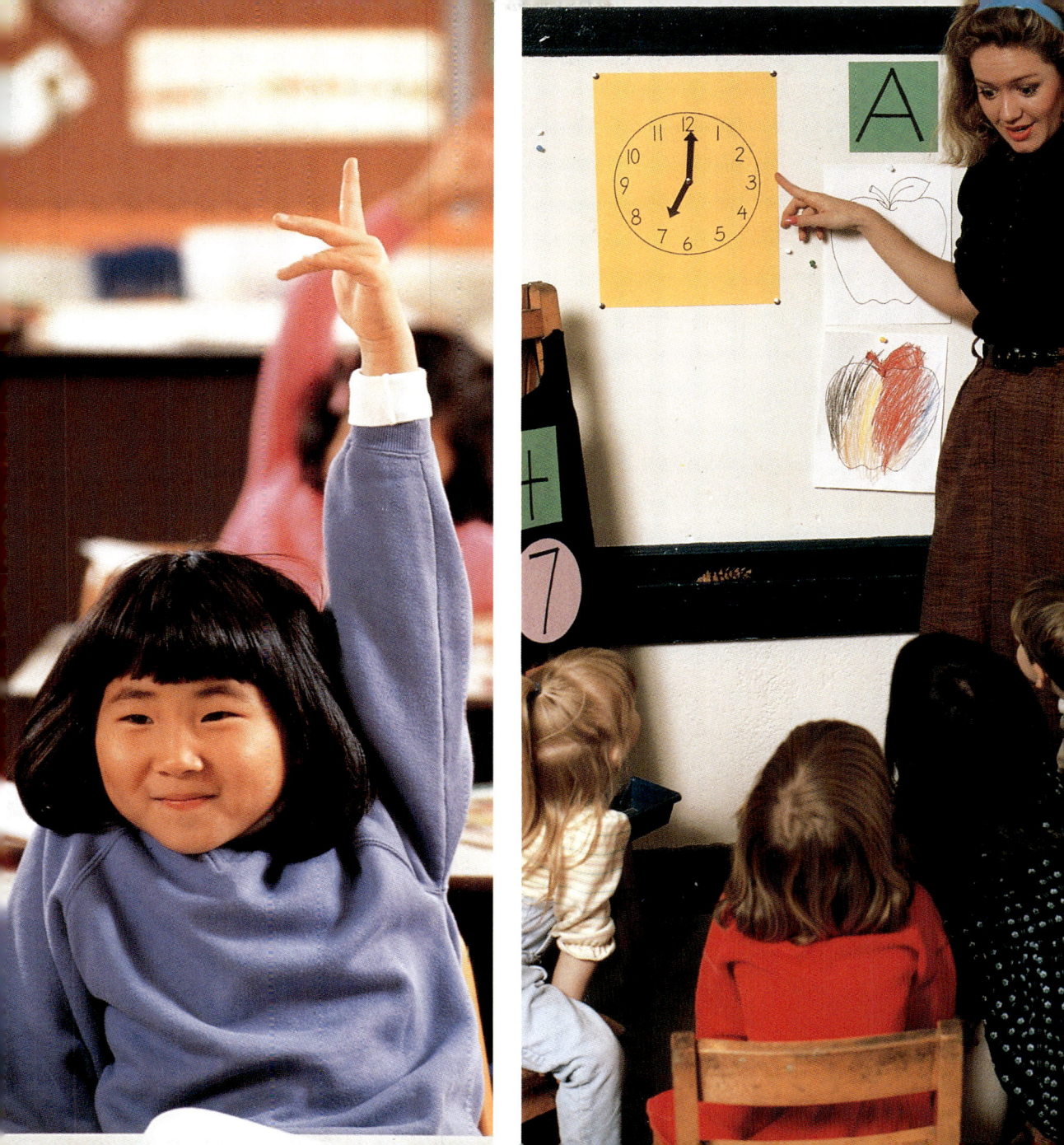

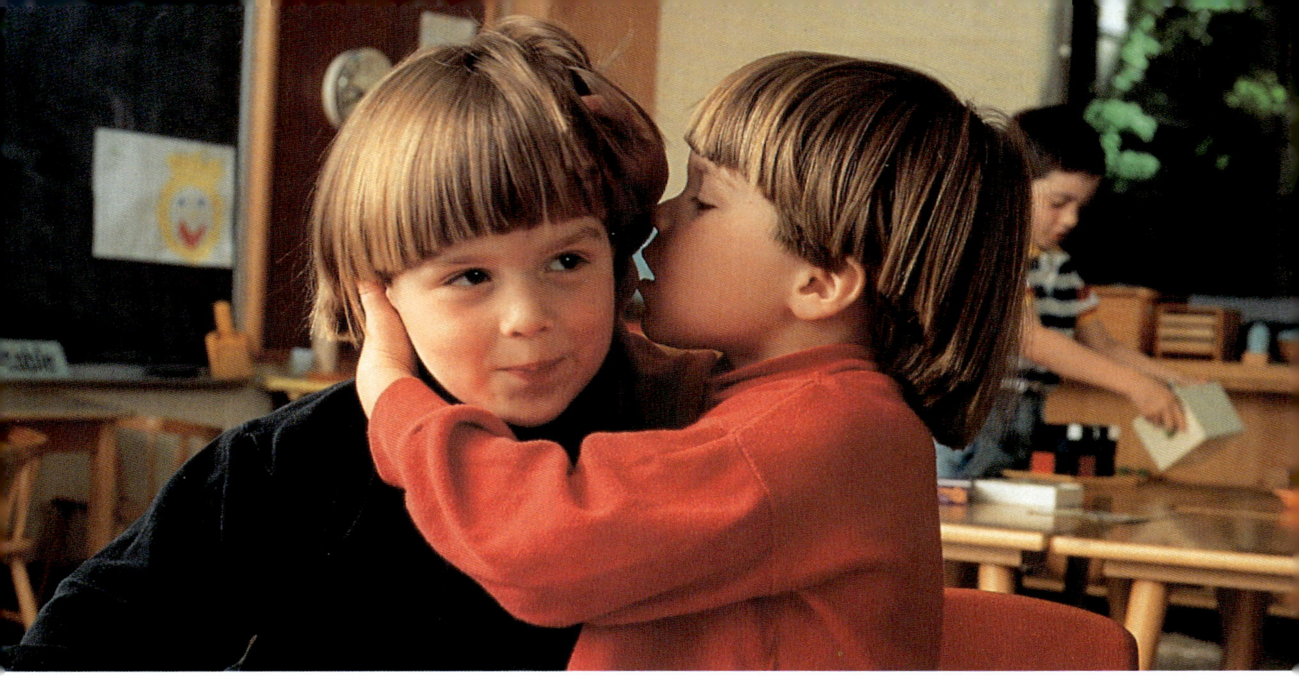

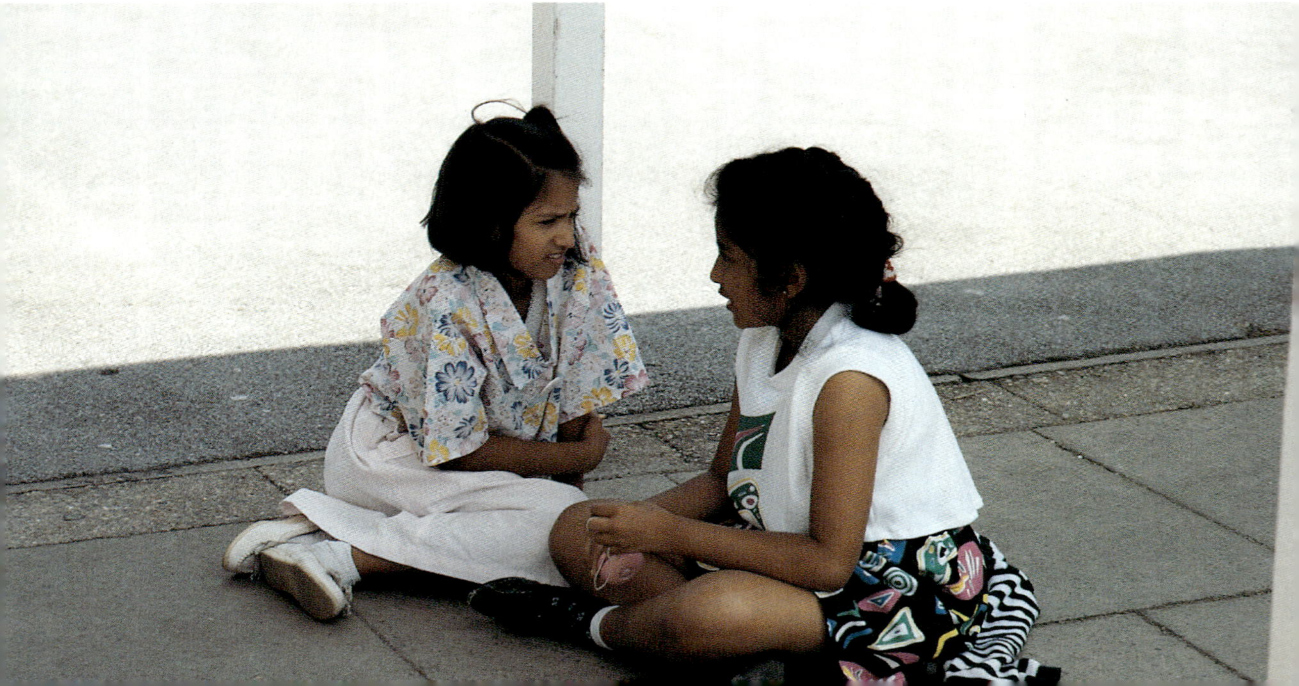

Talking to friends

By talking, you can share with
your friends. You can share
a joke, tell a secret, or discuss
your worries.

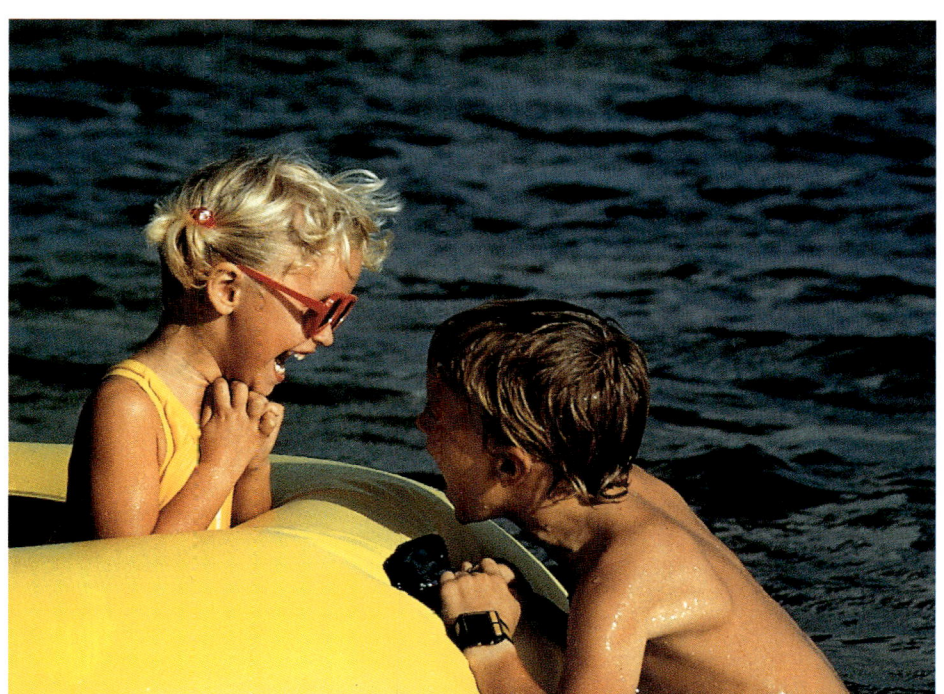

15

Learning together

The more you talk and listen,
discuss and examine things with
your friends, the more you learn
for yourself.

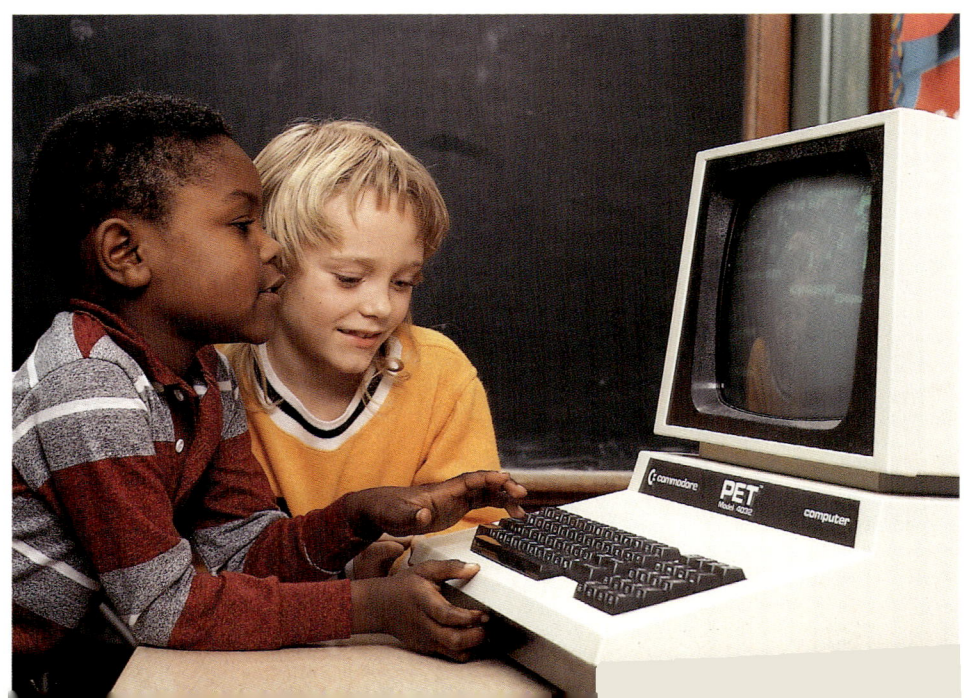

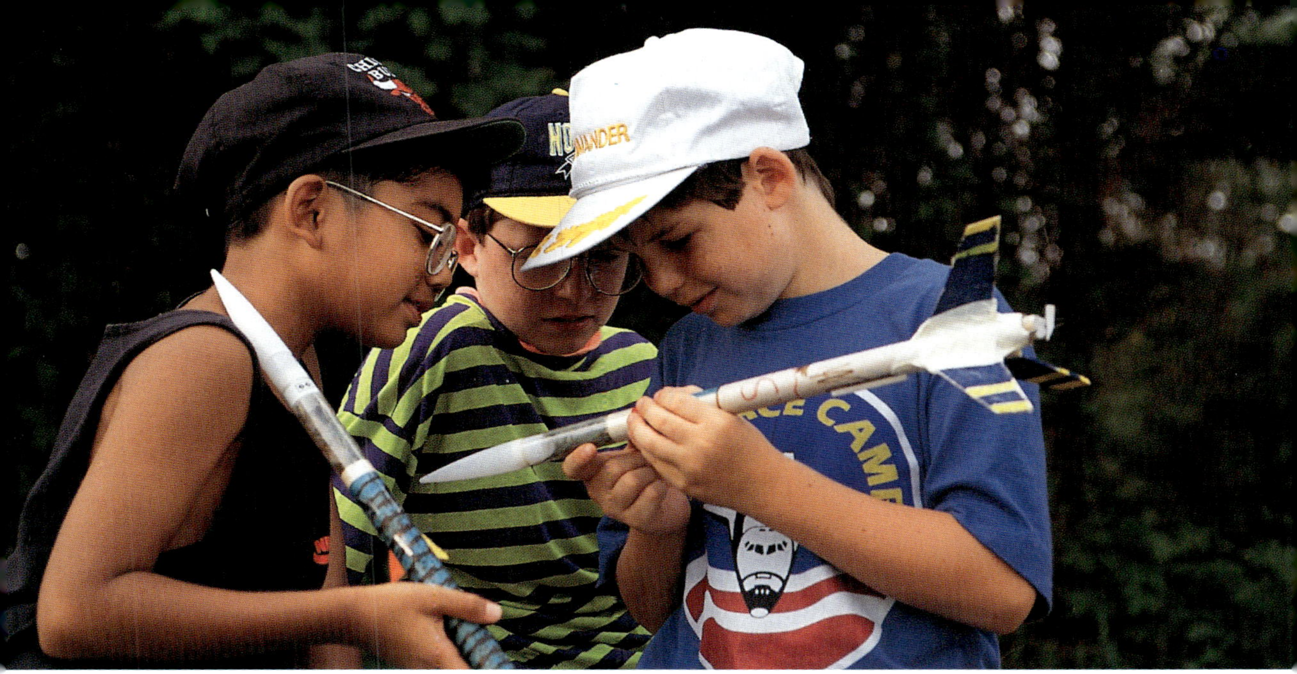

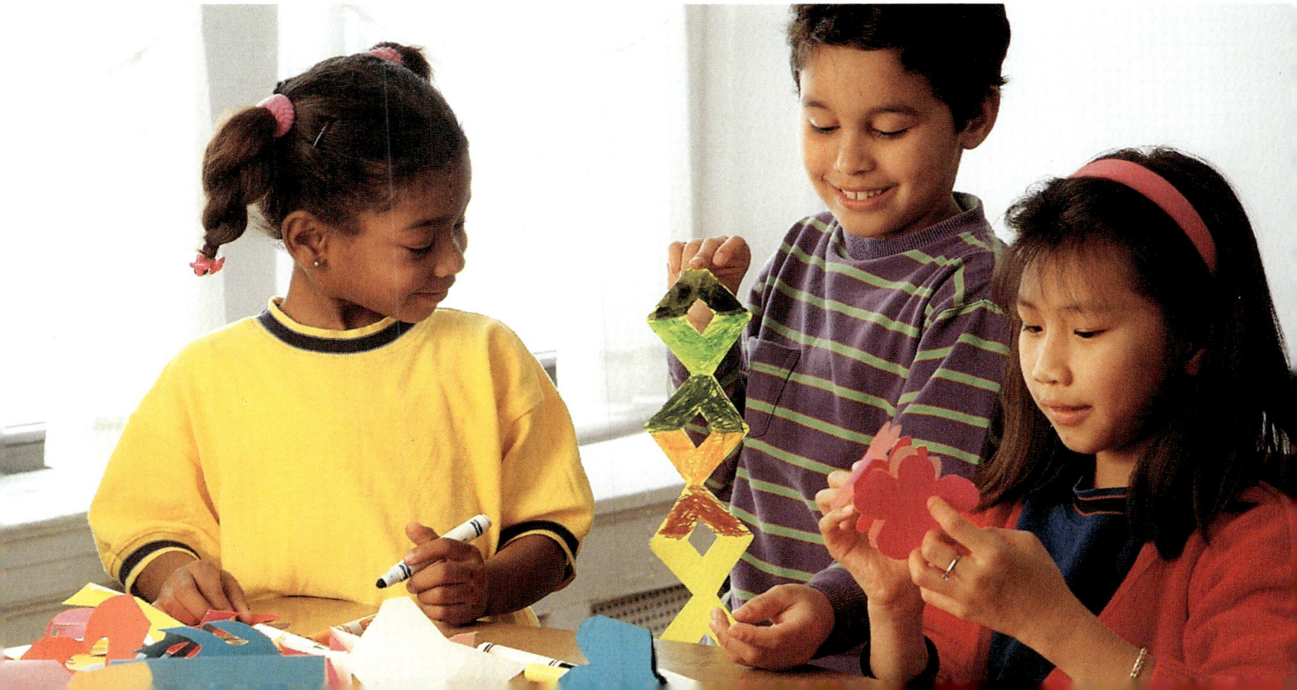

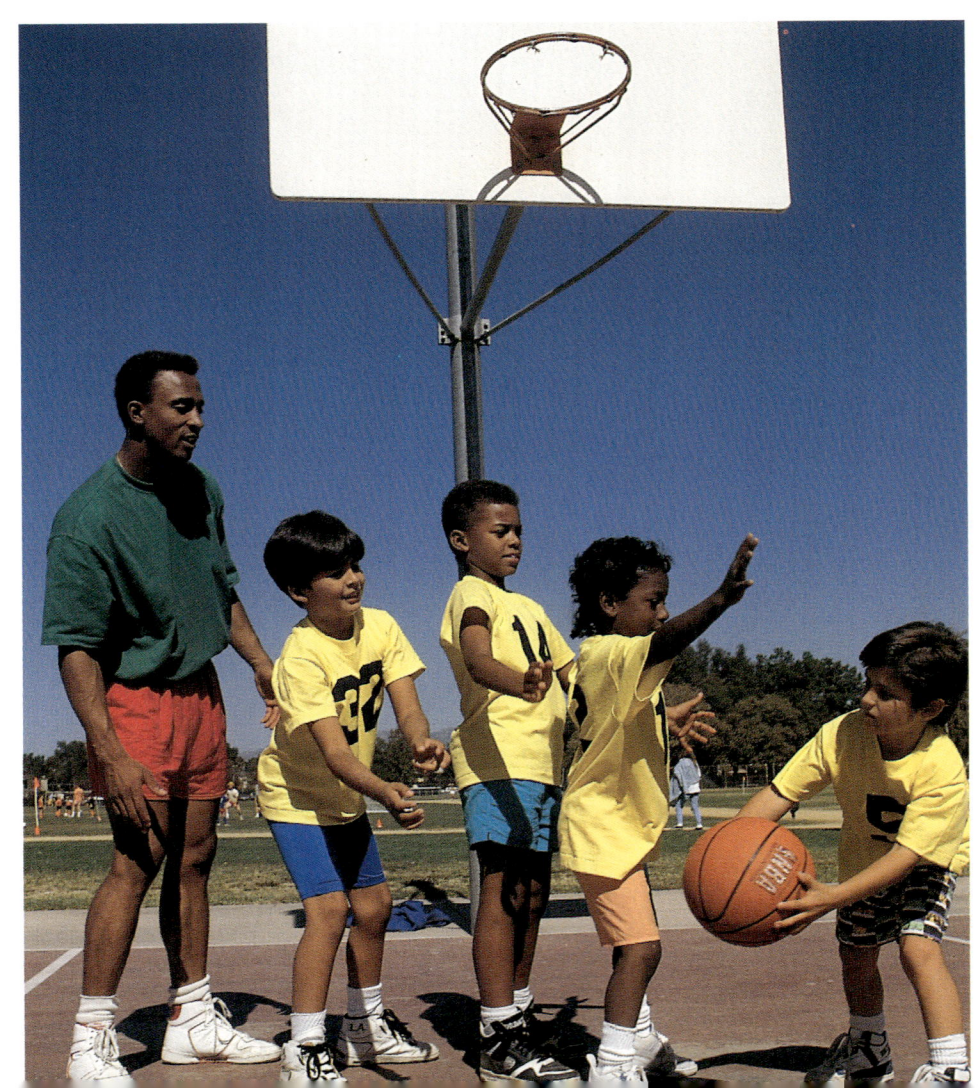

18

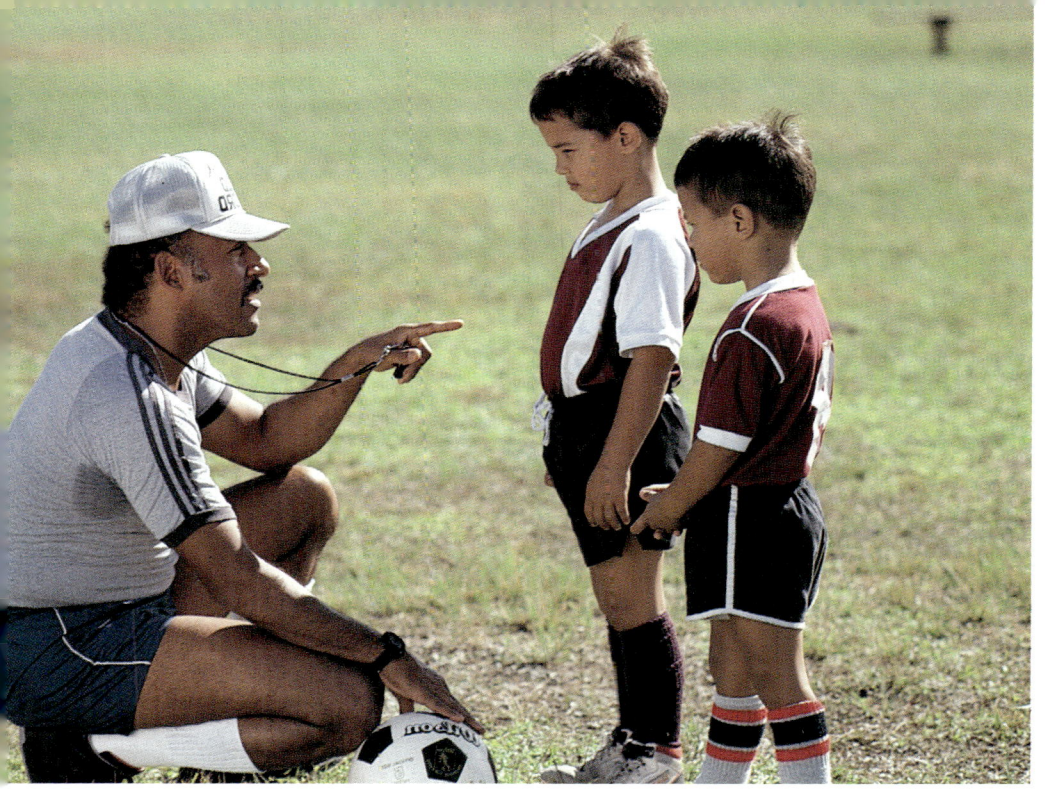

Learning a sport is great fun, but you need someone to help you. Someone to explain the best way.

How would you learn if talking was impossible?

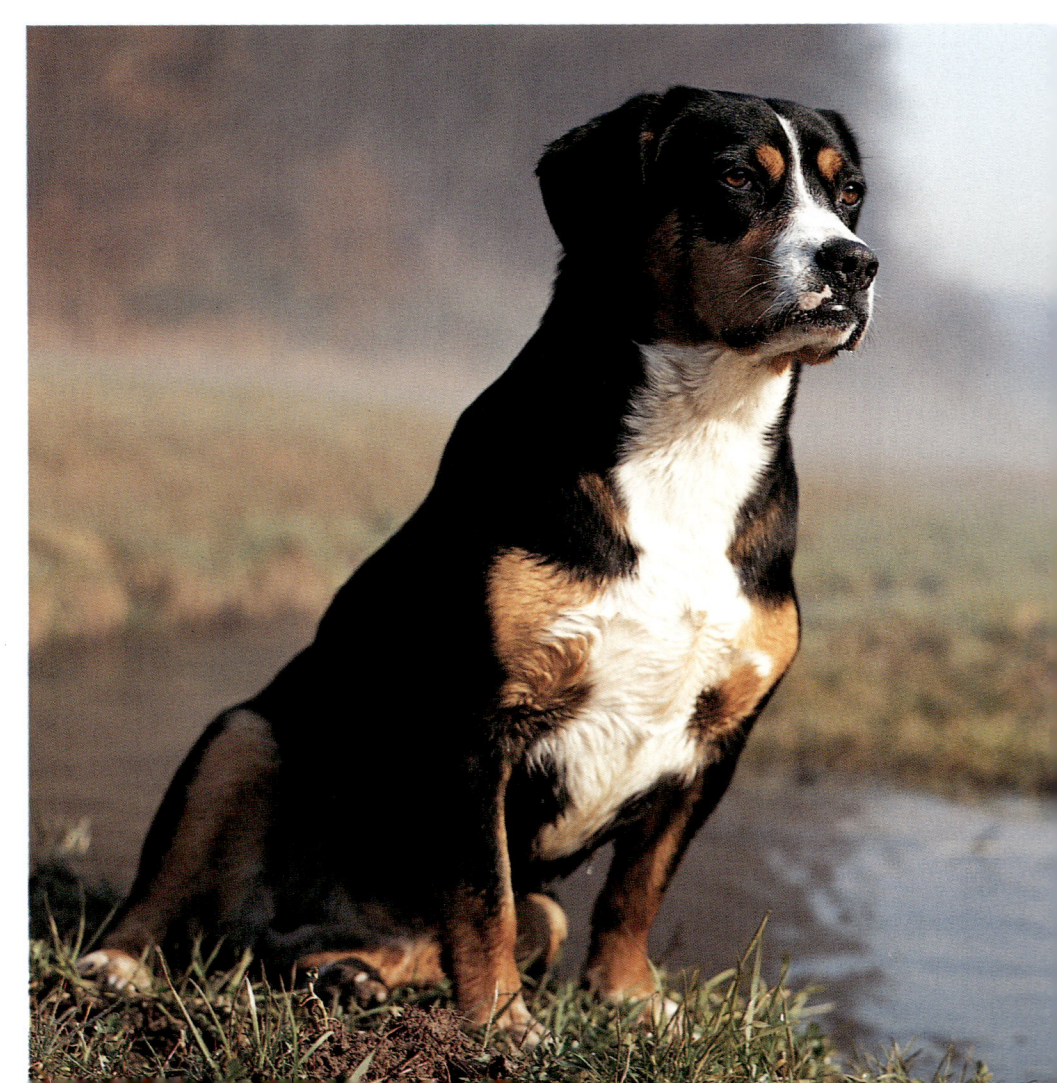

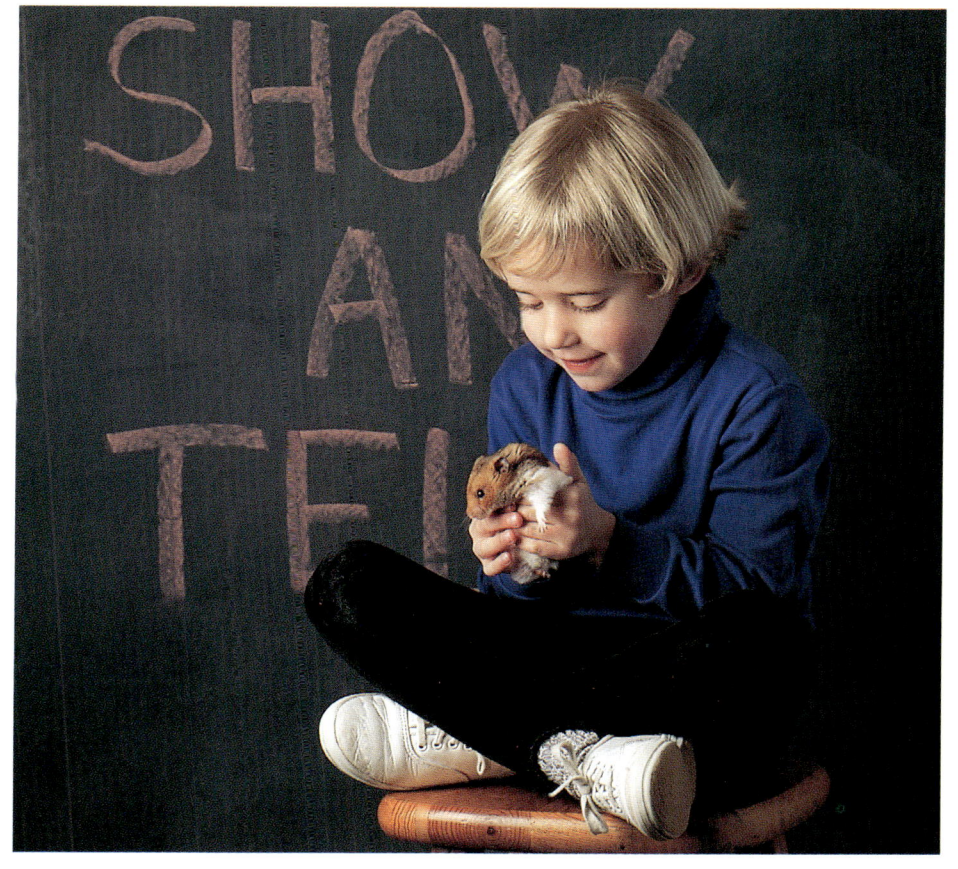

Animals like it when you to talk
to them. They don't understand
words, but they like the sound of
your voice. Dogs learn to 'sit'
when you say it in the right tone.

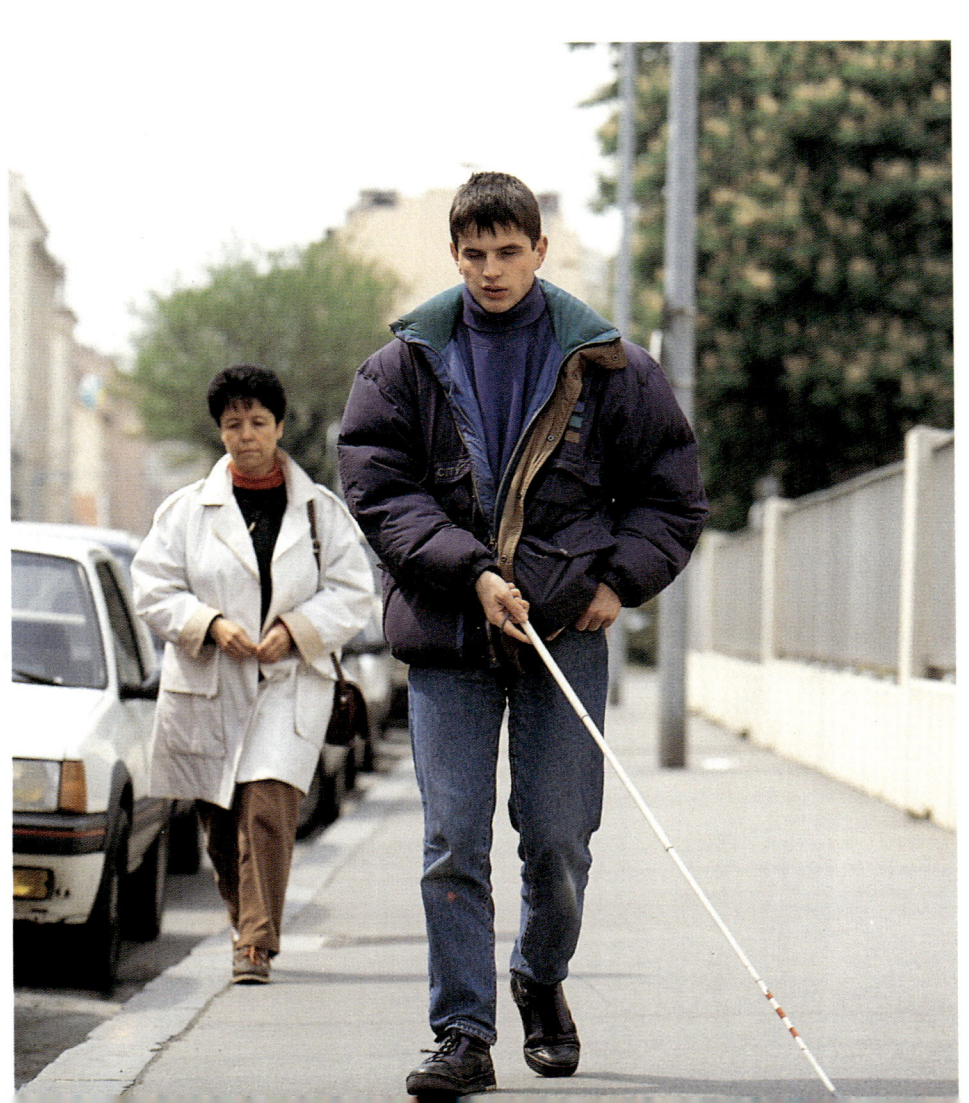

22

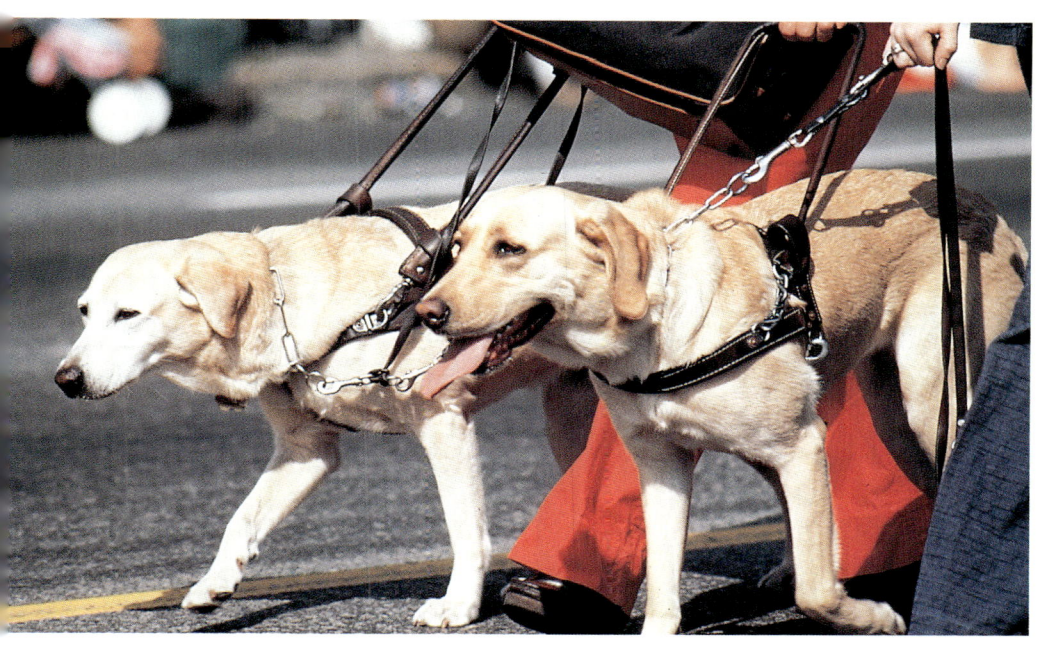

Blind people need help to learn
how to find their way around.
How do you think talking helps?

Guide dogs must learn too—they
learn voice signals and how to
behave in crowded places. 23

What if you're deaf?

Because they can't hear, deaf children find it difficult to learn to talk. They need special teaching.

They also need special teaching to learn lip-reading and sign-language.

Try covering your ears. Can you work out what people are saying from the way their lips move?

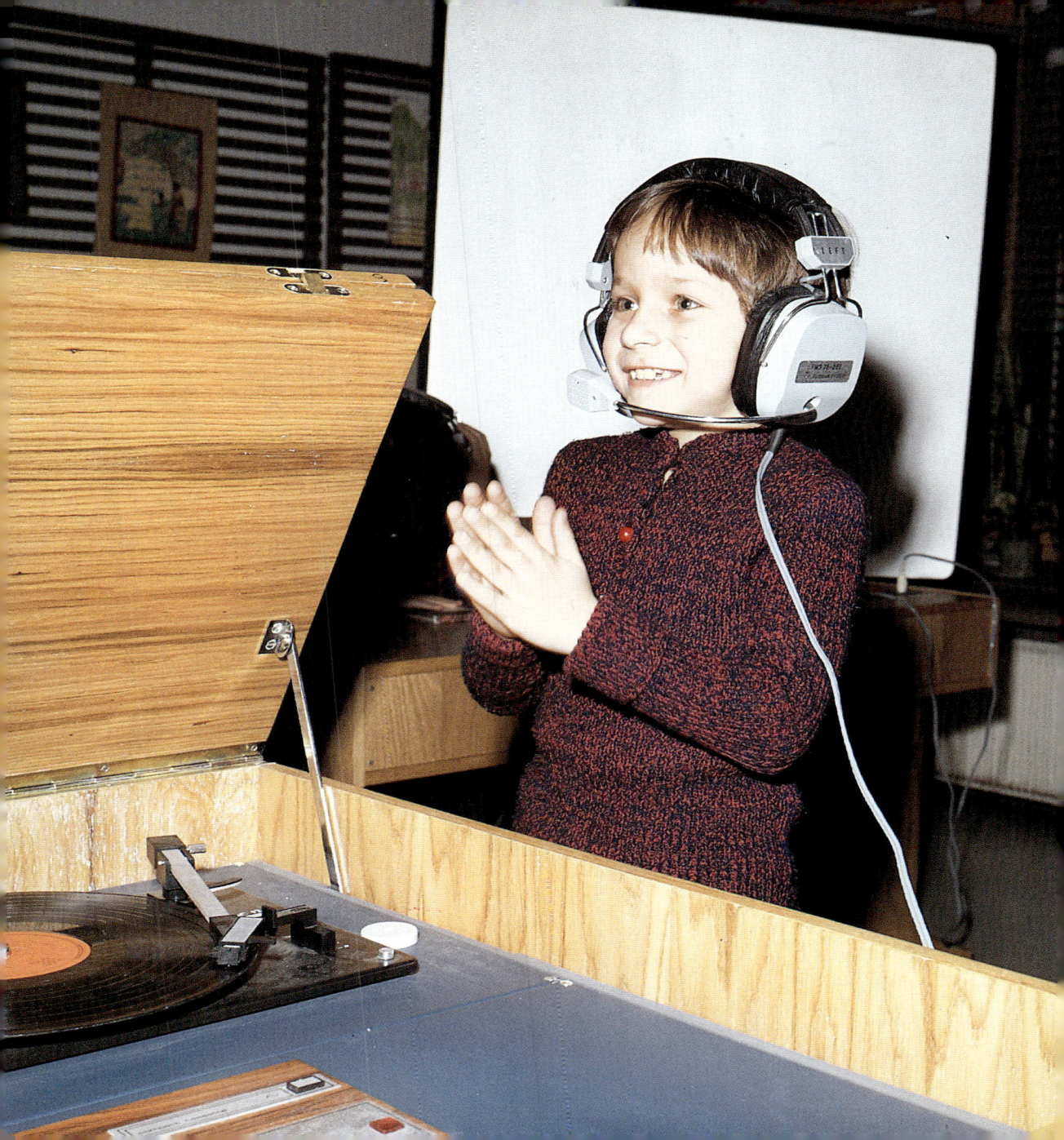

International Wildlife

ENGINEER
20

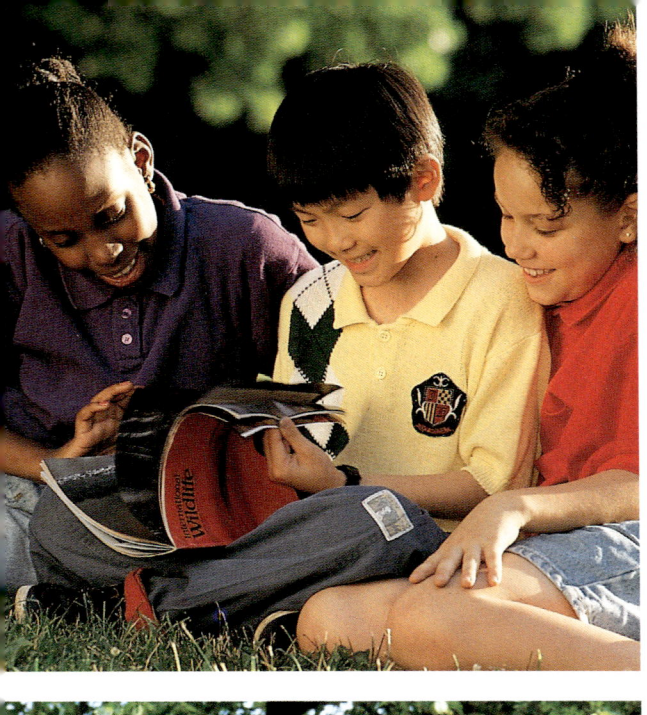

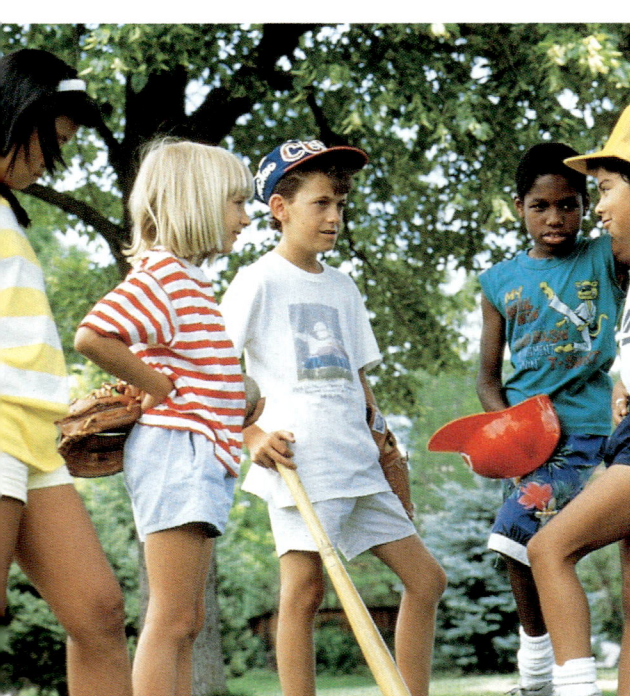

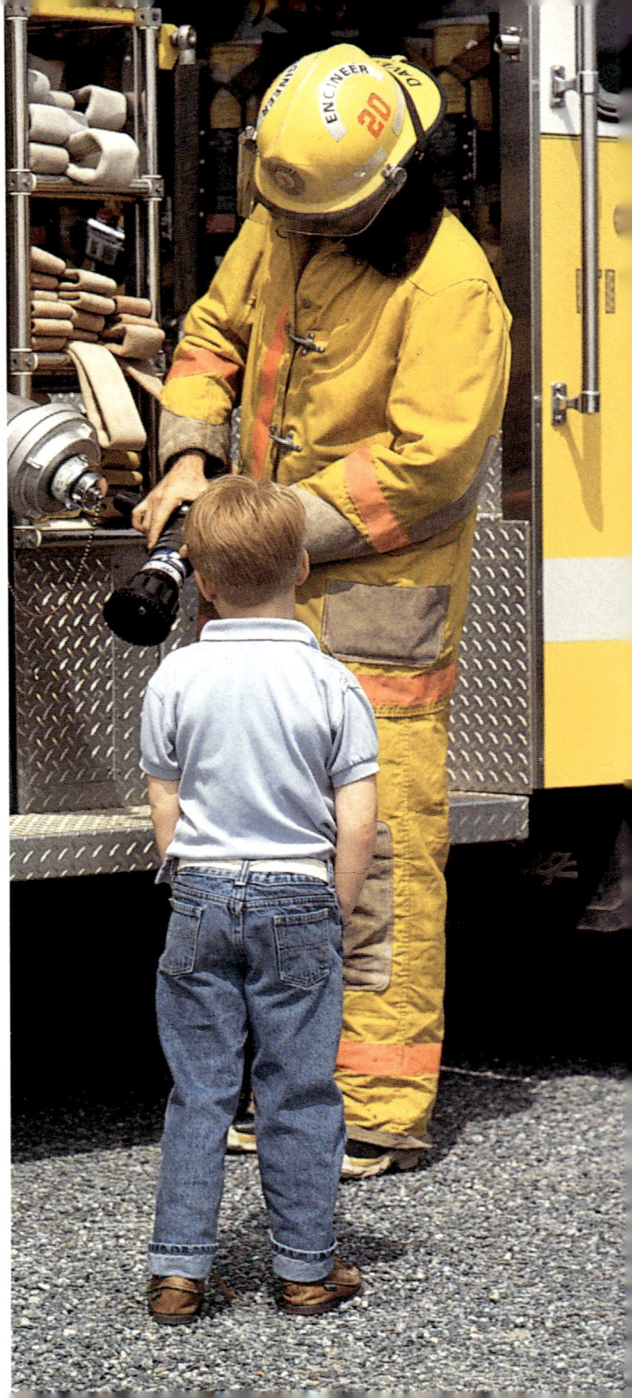

A skill for life

During your life you will need to talk to many different people for many different reasons.

You must learn how to hold a conversation—explain your feelings—give information—ask the right questions—and much, much more.

Talking is one of the most important skills you will ever learn.

communication Passing information from one person to another in any way—whether by talking, writing or making signals.

conversation
An exchange of
ideas by talking
together.

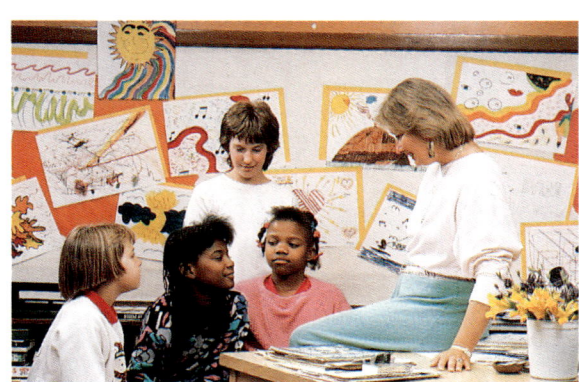

dumb Unable to speak.

lip-reading Understanding what people are saying by the way that their lips move.

28

sign-language A way of talking by making signals with the hands that is used by people who are deaf or dumb.

tone The quality of a sound—whether it is harsh or musical.

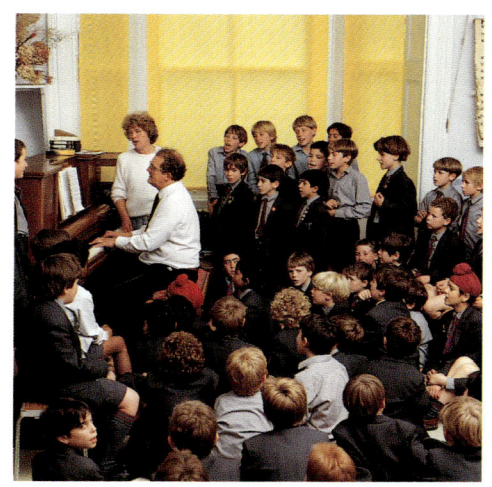

voice box The place in a person's throat where sounds are produced. The voice box contains chords of flesh which vibrate when air is forced past them.

29

Index